COPYRIGHT

Contents

Introduction

Thinking should be easy to do.

But most ordinary people find it hard to do.

Why?

Because they don't understand the context, environment, or framework in which they are operating in.

They don't understand the meaning or difference between of facts and assumptions.

It is my intent in this quick-read ebook to provide for the common man an easy to understand and power-pact way of thinking effectively and will allow your imagination to soar.

There will be no frills here, just insightful wisdom you can use today.

Thinking effectively is not easy due to multiple meanings of words by individuals based on culture and time. Trying to understand the culture and time(s) is important to understanding meaning.

Now, the foundation of thinking is knowing the five W's.

The questions are Who, What, When, Where, How, and Why.

When we read anything we should be looking to identify the answer to these questions.

The key here is not to identify the answers separately, but to identify the answers in combinations of twos (Who and What, When and Where, and How and Why?)

This technique gets you on the road to thinking effectively and faster.

Next you have to place the answers to those questions in the proper setting, environment, framework to establish a base of knowledge to be used as a reference point for future thoughts onto which you can link or relate to.

This provides the meaning.

Life consists of the past, present, and future.

The access to the past is our memory, access to the present is our senses, and access to the future is our imagination.

Of the three the most important should be your imagination.

Why?

Like Einstein said, "Imagination is more important than knowledge. Knowledge is limited. Imagination encircles the word."

Because even your memory is composed of imagination because you don't remember every detail of what happened, you fill in your thoughts with what you saw or felt was significant to you, thus imagined the things that you did not pay attention to.

Reread the last paragraph for it is important to understanding the importance of your imagination and how it can be used to create the success that you want in your life.

Now, it is our intent in this book have you put on Ph. D. Glasses that will allow you to see the deeper meanings of things; contextually and from a framework view.

We provide in this book a new formula that was discovered that can allow you to manifest good things that you desire in your life.

It is based upon the $E=MC^2$.

Second and finally we will provide to you a universal thinking process that you can use to learn billions of pieces of information.

Then we show you how to classify them into a easy to remember four step process that you see the relationship between different, dissimilar branches of knowledge, like philosophy, mathematics, music, and the sciences.

Two breakthrough things that can change your life lie ahead.

So let's get started.

Chapter 1 - E=MC^2

Curiosity will allow you to read and judge the focal point and how things are grouped around the point.

It will allow you to ask if there is a natural balance of resources?

What is the weight of the various components and will the foundations support them?

Center of Gravity Thinking

You will use Center of Gravity Thinking to learn how to know the difference between facts and opinion, how to obtain an accurate picture of existing conditions, and how to best use people, materials, machines and processes to maximize output with minimum waste of those resources.

Manifestation = Action / Center of Gravity of your Decision * Desire

Manifestation is equal to change of action divided by the center of gravity of your decision-making, which is influenced by your primary driver, which is fueled by curiosity.

In essence, curiosity drives your desire, desire drives your decision-making process, and your decisions drive your actions, which equals to manifestation.

Therefore, what you get in your life is determined by how curious you are about things around you.

It is a simple formula, yet truth is revealed in it.

Clausewitz's and My Thoughts On Center of Gravity and The Future.

There must be a move to develop your thinking using the concept of center of gravity.

You have to determine your decision points and vulnerabilities in order to solve the current problems.

A look at a leading authority shows how Claude Von Clausewitz viewed center of gravity.

Clausewitz felt that center of gravity is the concentration of combat power. He felt that at every level of war there is a different center of gravity.

Strategic examples according to Clausewitz are a nation's capital, a city, its leaders or even public opinion.

Center of gravity is the relevant mass of your power that is made significant by your corresponding will to use it.

Center of gravity is the derivative of the aims or objectives established at the level you are planning.

Not all sources of strength are center of gravities...

Clausewitz says that every level of war has a different center of gravity.

One must determine the center of gravity first at each level, beginning at the quantum level.

He says that one can find the enemy center of gravity where the concentration of combat power is, it is always found where the mass is concentrated most densely.

It is vital to accomplish his aims.

At the end of the day, we must move away from theories about center of gravity when we consider various scenarios and probe into the reality basis of center of gravities.

Center of gravity is the derivative of the aims or objectives established at the level you are planning.

One must submit each potential center of gravity to a validity test. If one desires to impose his will upon a center of gravity, will that action create a cascading deteriorating effect on morale, cohesion and will to fight that prevents the enemy from achieving his aims and allows the achievement of our own?

If I have a valid center of gravity, do I have a feasible ability to impose my will over it?

If I cannot, or not completely, consider an- other potential center of gravity .

Center of gravities are dynamic and may change as the conflict.

The strategic level is dominant in the continuum of war because it is at this level that the political, economic, military and other aims are defined and thus the importance of planning from the top down.

Aims must be determined.

The aim and the resources allocated to achieve that aim is intimately linked.

Center of gravity of resources is the essence of his resources enabling him to achieve results.

So the formula for manifestation is:

Manifestation = Action / Center of Gravity of your Decision * Desire

Remember manifestation is equal to action taken divided by the center of gravity of your decisions, which is influenced by your primary driver, which is fueled by curiosity.

In essence, curiosity drives your desire, desire drives your decision-making process, and your decisions drive your actions, which equals to manifestation.

Therefore, what you get in your life is determined by how curious you are about things around you.

See and understand the next statements and you will be well on your way to success in life.

Curiosity will allow you to read and judge the focal point and how things are grouped around the point.

It will allow you to ask if there is a natural balance of resources?

What is the weight of the various components and will the foundations support them?

It is a simple formula, yet truth is revealed in it.

We must be able to see across the full spectrum of thinking and decisions in order to increase efficiency and using the critical thinking as a tool that is and will be a measurement for the foreseeable future.

Now that you have manifested your reality, we will now take a look at how you can operate in the manifested (real) world and use a smart technique that will allow you to learn information quicker.

Chapter 2 - Ph. D. Glasses

Facts and assumptions resulting from the mission analysis are measured against a framework of four functional areas.

Facts are statements of known data concerning the situation.

Many people have a problem identifying facts or just ignore facts because they don't' know how to properly apply them.

You should focus on the "so what" of the fact.

You say to yourself, here is a fact and what does this fact mean?

Is the fact a cause or effect, what are the pros or cons, is it a general to specific fact or specific to general fact, is the factual relationship a numerical or historical context?

A fact is real whether you it is known or unknown.

If a fact is known, you can measure it.

If it is unknown, you can measure it by use of statistical probability of what you think you would see or where it is suppose to be located, or it could be an assumption.

Assumptions are suppositions or unknowns about the current or future situation, which are assumed true in the absence of facts, and are required to continue planning.

Assumptions should not wish away capabilities or assume capabilities.

Your biggest enemy will be the unknown and assumptions.

All assumptions not validated or eliminated in planning become risks in execution.

This captures all that planners currently know and don't know in an easily referenced format.

Next, be careful to build the framework in which you will leverage and execute your tasks.

The framework gives you boundaries from which you will operate within.

Here you determine what right looks like in the future.

If you can't see in the future, you can't take action and execute your power.

Frameworks allow you to focus key people by identifying tasks, deciding what's important and what to measure and how to measure it, and at what acceptable risk to determine if you need help to achieve your desired results.

The following is a **Four (4) Step Framework** for you to use as you go through the decision making process.

As part of the process, the five basic questions you should always be able to ask and answer are:

1.   Where are you currently located?

2.   Why are you there?

3.   How do you support from there?

4.   How do you get support from there?

5.   When, to where, and in what sequence do you move to ensure continuous operations?

These 4 steps are based on the customer and the customer's needs.

You should address the following when analyzing a task:

(supported organization or who are you supporting) = **requirements**,

(supporting organization or who are you supporting) = **capabilities**

(what is your ability to support and who is supporting you) = **standards**, and **timeline**.

These steps can be used throughout the decision-making process to make your best decision.

They will allow you to "sense" or measure success, have wide visibility: connectivity 24/7 of data architecture, global focus.

"Control" things by having Unit of Effort: Right people and capabilities, shared awareness and processes, same standards of success, and to "Respond" to issues with Rapid & Precise Response: Speed, Reliability, Visibility, Efficiency.

In this quick-read are the tools you need to become a millionaire, some even a billionaire because it will allow you to go beyond your current abilities to process information.

Other books/programs that you might enjoy...

Today, you can get my best selling book, "Master the Art of Context Thinking" at www.etsy.com and www.etsy.com/listing/ 176998568/master-the-art-of-context-thinking?.

About the Author

Dr. Joseph W. Graham, Ph. D., Business Administration, BS in Graphic Design. He served in Operation Desert Storm, Operation Restore Democracy in Haiti, and Operation Enduring and Iraqi Freedom. His highest military award is the Bronze Star Medal.

He's known as one of the world's unified thinkers and founder of a breakthrough thinking method called Context Thinking.

www.contextthinking.com

He is also founder of *The Super-Elite Thinking Series.*

Full Professional Biography

A 10-year veteran of the context thinking field, Joseph Graham is unique among experts as the man who's actually developed and executed the day-to-day thinking strategies.

Today, he's the #1 best selling author of *Master The Art of Context Thinking, The 11 Golden Principles of Context Thinking, Sense & Respond: Thinking at a 24/7 Pace, Thinking Quadrant: How to Think on Your Feet Even When You're Sitting, Rapid Perception*, and many others, published worldwide.

Dr. Graham speaks annually to entrepreneurs, independent sales professionals, corporate employees and industry association members on the principles of context thinking.

As one of America's most respected authorities in the knowledge products industry, he also helps achievers who are experts in their field attain worldwide status and million- dollar incomes by developing their thinking around their business strategies, training concepts, industry expertise and unique market posture using context thinking.

Dr. Graham lives in Columbia, South Carolina. Other information can be found at www.contextthinking.com.

You can take online classes:

Online Critical Thinking Course for Instructors, Executives, Military Personnel, Nursing, College Students, Adult Education, and Others

Learn the foundations of **Integrated Critical Active Thinkin**g while incorporating them into your classes/ profession.

Sessions: Open Now!

JGraham Enterprises, LLC, Founder of Context Thinking Courses will be offering for individuals interested in developing their understanding of integrated critical active thinking and their ability to bring it into the foundation of instruction.

Non-Academic Credit

(Registration limited to 15 Students per class session).

ONLINE REGISTRATION IS NOW OPEN

Registration fees include costs for all instructional materials. Instructional materials for each course can be accessed upon signup at www.learnopia.com for the course.

http://www.learnopia.com/course/icat/

The Complete Online Learning Solution

Learnopia is a learning management system (LMS) where you register for our online courses. Students through dis- tance education classes can learn new skills for their career.

The purpose of our online course is to provide individuals of any subject or field the opportunity to acquire an in- depth, hands-on understanding of how to use the tools of integrated critical active thinking as the basis for planning, instruction, and learning.

Dr. Joseph Graham has ten years experience in using con- text and critical thinking, Dr. Graham brings a wealth of experience to the integrated critical active thinking and context thinking online courses. Recognizing the importance of placing critical and context thinking at the heart of instruction,

Dr. Graham took a systematic approach to bringing critical and context thinking into practice.

He holds a Ph.D., MBA, BBA in Business Administration and a BS in Graphic Design.

What are the course costs?

The basic course cost, for each course, Non-academic credit, is $35.

Register right away, approximately 15 students per course. Registration is now open for the course.

Registration fees include costs for all instructional materials. Instructional materials for each course can be accessed upon signup at www.learnopia.com for the course.

Course Description iCAT: Introduction to Integrated Critical Active Thinking

Introduces the theory and application of critical thinking. It fosters understanding of how to learn critical thinking skills to students for any subject, discipline. In this course, you will

Questions

How does the integrated critical active thinking online course work?

The course will deepen your understanding of critical thinking while you are working it in your specific profession.

Once registered for the course, you can log in at any time. You may look through the tools within the site and read the books and listen to any videos on the site.

Who will be teaching the courses?

The courses are taught by Dr. Joseph Graham, who has years of experience as well as a deep understanding of the basics of integrated critical active thinking to effectively bring critical thinking into instruction. Dr. Graham uses innovative tools for online course delivery.